Baby Making Machine

How to Get Pregnant Fast and Easy

By Sly V Marko

Notice

By purchasing this book you agree with the following: You understand that the information contained on this page and this book is an opinion, and should be used for the purposes of entertainment only.

You are responsible for your own behavior and none of this book should be consider legal or personal advice.

Dedication

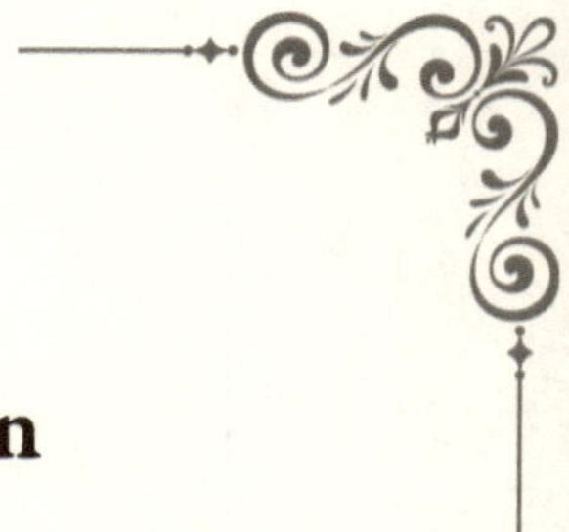

I dedicate this book to anyone who desires to have a baby but have been finding it difficult.

I trust that after going through this book, you will get pregnant with your own child

Introduction

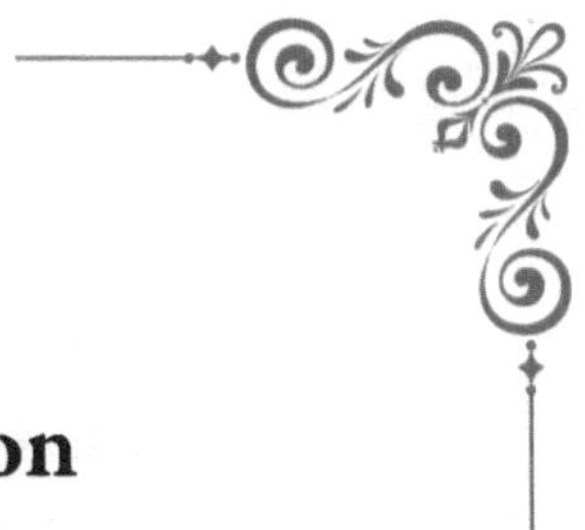

Everyone loves babies, especially if they are from our own tummy.

I UNDERSTAND THAT NOT every woman gets pregnant easily, there might be one problem or the other stopping you from conceiving.

BUT I BELIEVE THAT what we have to share with you will go a long way in helping you get your own baby.

SO READ THIS BOOK WITH rapt attention and test some of the methods outlined. You are free to run them by your physician.

GOOD LUCK.

How Your Sexual Positions Plays An Certain Role When You Want to Get Pregnant

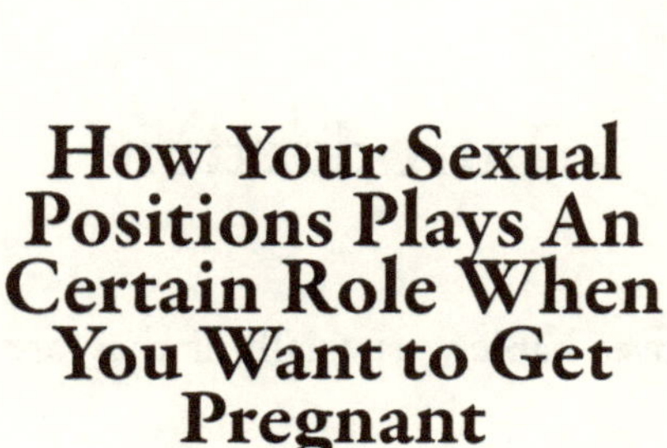

It is probably the simplest thing in the entire world; however there are certain couples who are unable to conceive for certain reasons which could be inclusive of scarce or else feeble sperm count.

WHEN YOU ARE LEARNING the process on how to get pregnant, there are times in which both you and your better half could necessitate a thrust in the right direction which would significantly augment your chances of getting pregnant.

WHEN YOU ARE DETERMINING the ideal position to amplify your chances of getting pregnant, remember that the standard policy is that it is essential for the male sperm to be placed as close to to the female cervix as feasible. This is the essential norm which aids in conception.

THIS IS DEPENDENT ON the life term of the male sperm as well as the female egg. As soon as the egg is freed from the ovary it is a stage which is also popular as ovulation, thereby the process is initiated when it commences its pathway downward from the fallopian tube all the way till it reaches its ultimate aim which is the uterus.

An unrestricted egg normally stays alive for 24 hours, whereas it is possible for a sperm to last anyplace beginning three to five days inside the feminine body.

IT IS A RULE THAT THE egg has to be as near to the sperm as it is feasible to do so, subsequent to which they can assemble and fasten together prior to the egg's demise.

THERE ARE LOTS OF PEOPLE who opine that the sexual positions have no relation with the process of getting pregnant.

THE LOGICAL CONCLUSION which can be arrived at is that it is sensible to form the position which would assist in the process wherein the sperm congregates with the egg and this process is initiated within the shortest probable time span.

THIS IS EVEN MORE SO for people who have quite a problem when it comes to conceiving and have been trying so, ineffectively for quite some time.

THE INITIAL POSITION which is necessitated when you wish to get pregnant is to stay away from positions that ensure the slightest rendering of the cervix to the male sperm, as well as positions which commonly resist gravity like sex which is initiated while sitting down, or with the woman on top or else when you are standing up.

Also bear in mind that when you are in the midst of conceiving, it is advisable if you can ensure that you restrict the quantity of sperm which is permitted to travel back from the vagina.

When you are ascertaining the process on how to get pregnant, bear in mind that it is mandatory that the woman's hips must necessarily be placed in a way which would make it feasible for the sperm which is unconfined to be kept within, which would ensure that it has adequate time within which it is capable of spinning up to the cervix.

THIS IS HOW SEXUAL positions would assist you when you are ascertaining how to get pregnant.

How To Get Pregnant By Modifying Your Lifestyle

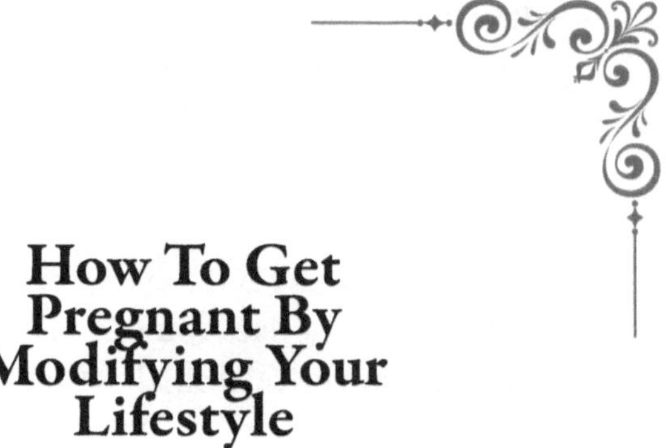

While some women are blessed with fertility, others find it quite difficult to get pregnant. In case you are one belonging to the latter group you would know how frustrating it is to keep on trying.

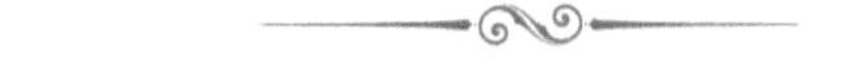

HOWEVER, MOST OF THE times this process are made frustrating further because of the lack of knowledge that comes with it. Most of the times people do not take all the measures that are necessary to get pregnant.

THAT IS EXACTLY WHY you should not only do you research well as to how to get pregnant, but you will have to ensure that you take all the steps that are possible for you to get pregnant.

THE FIRST WAY TO ENSURE that you get pregnant is by having unprotected sex during ovulation. For this you would have to ensure when you are ovulating.

GENERALLY OVULATION takes effect on the 13th or the 14th day of menstrual cycle. You can easily determine this day by using an ovulation calculator. These are easily available in the regular drugstores.

YOU COULD ALSO PURCHASE a basal body thermometer, which again helps you determine your ovulating date. To increase chances of getting pregnant start having regular unprotected sex around 2 days before your actual ovulation date.

HOWEVER, THAT IS NOT the only way on how to get pregnant. You should also at the same time take a lot of steps to modify your lifestyle and dietary pattern.

THE BEGINNING STEP is to modify your diet. Ensure that you are cutting down as much as possible on the junk food that you have and try to incorporate a balanced diet in your food intake.

ENSURE THAT YOU ARE taking all the vitamins that you need to take. You should also include lots of fresh food and water.

It is a myth that good dietary habits are meant to be treated during pregnancy. In fact you should begin taking a healthy diet way before you even conceive.

YOU SHOULD ALSO GIVE up on all your bad health habits if you have any. In case you are heavily into consuming alcohol, you should stop immediately. Smoking is another health choice that does not go well with pregnancy.

YOU WOULD HAVE TO QUIT smoking, drinking and doing drugs. This is not just in respect to women who are trying to get pregnant but, her partner should also quit any habits if he has any.

IN FACT STUDIES HAVE shown that these habits interfere with the sperm count and thus lessening the chance of getting pregnant. When you are reading on how to get pregnant, it is quite important to keep the man's perspective in view.

TO BETTER YOUR CHANCES even further, it is a good idea to take prenatal vitamins that are available in the drugstores.

These help in increasing the chances of pregnancy and also ensure the health of the child, once conceived.

HOWEVER, IT IS EXPEDIENT that you consult a physician before having these pills. It is indeed important to modify your lifestyle before you get pregnant.

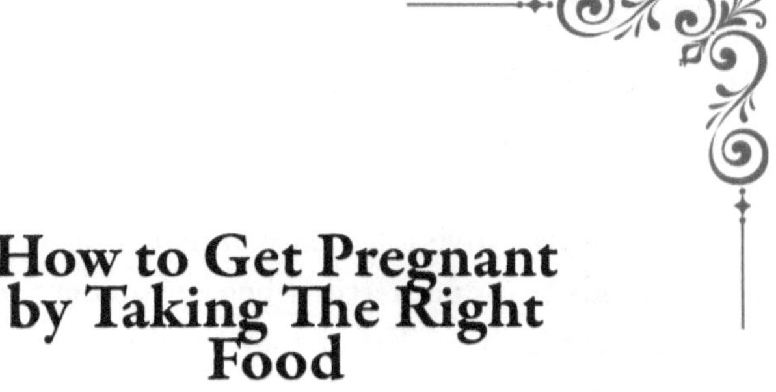

How to Get Pregnant by Taking The Right Food

Are you tired of trying with no results? Do you feel that your body is letting you down in one of the most important wishes of your life? In case you are then do not give up so soon.

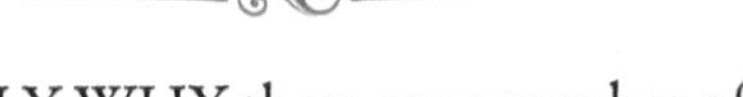

THERE ARE MANY COUPLES who face problems in conceiving at the right time. One of the major reasons behind this is the lifestyle that we lead. Since we have pushed our normal age of child bearing further, it becomes quite difficult for us to conceive when we really want to.

THAT IS EXACTLY WHY there are a number of couples who are trying their level best to lay their hands upon the right tips on how to get pregnant.

THERE ARE MANY WAYS and tips that are available on how to get pregnant. While some of the tips are completely natural there are many artificial techniques as well.

OF COURSE TO INCREASE their chances for pregnancy there are many couples who pick to follow the artificial as well as natural techniques of getting pregnant.

It is however advisable that you first concentrate on the natural methods to induce fertility before you have to take recourse to the synthetic ones. The artificial techniques of getting pregnant provide you with lower guarantee and are often quite costly as well.

IF YOU ASK ANYONE ON how to get pregnant naturally the obvious answer would be to have unprotected sex during ovulation. Yet it is true that there are loads of couples out there who do take all the care to track their ovulation with no success.

THAT IS BECAUSE THERE are many women who lose their fertility quotient due to the various stress and strains of modern day living.

SO IN CASE YOU ARE one of these women you must be wondering how to get pregnant by increasing the fertility quotient of your body?

The best and most obvious solution to this answer to how to get pregnant is the right diet. It is certainly very important for you to follow the right diet to get your body working the right way. Unless your body is in the best of the health the hormones of your body would not function in the best way.

THERE ARE A NUMBER of diet supplement that are available which would allow you to get the right kind of hormone function.

In fact there are loads of prenatal vitamins supplement present which can induce pregnancy. Other food supplements like Zinc and calcium are also good for the fertility of the body.

ANOTHER EXCELLENT DIETARY supplement that could be used to induce fertility in the body is soy isoflavone. Now the most important question is how to get pregnant using soy isoflavone?

THE TRICK IS TO TAKE right amounts of these at the right time. The best time to have these is the 3rd to 5th day of your menstrual cycle.

THIS WOULD MEAN THE 3rd day from the first day of your period. As far as the quantity is concerned it is best to consult a dietician or a gynecologist. Taking the appropriate food at the right time multiplies your chances of getting pregnant.

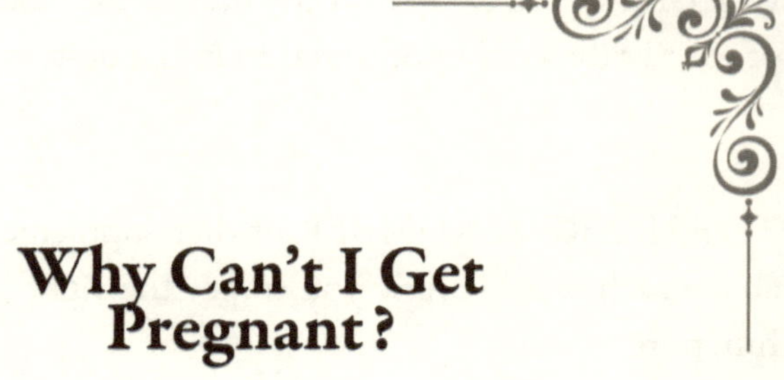

Why Can't I Get Pregnant?

One of the useful suggestions you can give to any women to get pregnant is to have sex. One of the most common question among women is "Why can not I get pregnant"?

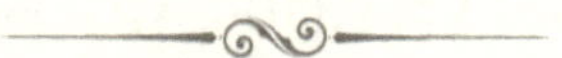

NOWADAYS A LOT OF WOMEN consider they'll be pregnant the moment they leave the pill, but in reality, it's not that simple. Time is another important factor, which plays a significant role to get pregnant. To increase your chances of conceiving quickly, women need a bit of calculations.

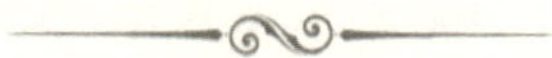

MAKE SURE TO HAVE SEX at the peak level of your ovulation cycle. Its is the most fertile period of your menstrual cycle and during that period you can double your chances of getting pregnant by having sex at that time.

THERE ARE NUMEROUS techniques that you can apply to find out the exact time of your ovulation cycle. The finest way to check out the peak time to conceive a baby is an ovulation kit.

This kit assists you to make a chart of your body's temperature. As charting, the accurate time of peak fertility is the key to get pregnant.

A LOT OF WOMEN ALSO use an ovulation calendar that graphs the time since their last menstrual cycle. The normal cycle comprises of 28 days, and typically 14th day or 12 – 16th is the peal of ovulation and perhaps the best time to have sex with your partner.

A LOT OF COUPLES THINK the best and fastest formula to conceive is to have intercourse all the time. This is wrong approach. When a male does intercourse frequently, it reduces the sperm count. A lower sperm count means lower probability of fertilization.

THE BEST STRATEGY TO conceive is to take at least 48hr rest between two meetings. One can try his chance three times a week during ovulation cycle.

SOMETIMES MALES COME up with an idea of saving their sperms for one big short. This is ridiculous and insane idea to follow or think of following.

AFTER 72 HOURS, YOUR sperms will become slow, deformed and lethargic. The best way to keep your sperm pool healthy and fresh is to have intercourse after every 48hr.

THEREFORE, KEEP IN mind excessive sex act will only reduce your efficiency and sperm count. Most couples lack scientific knowledge about ovulation cycle and try to get pregnant by chance. One good option is to take support from ultrasound and other latest sonography techniques.

AN ULTRASOUND GRAPH tells you your exact ovulation time and increases the chances of getting pregnant. My final piece of advice is to keep your sperm count healthy and have sex on every alternative day for a couple on months.

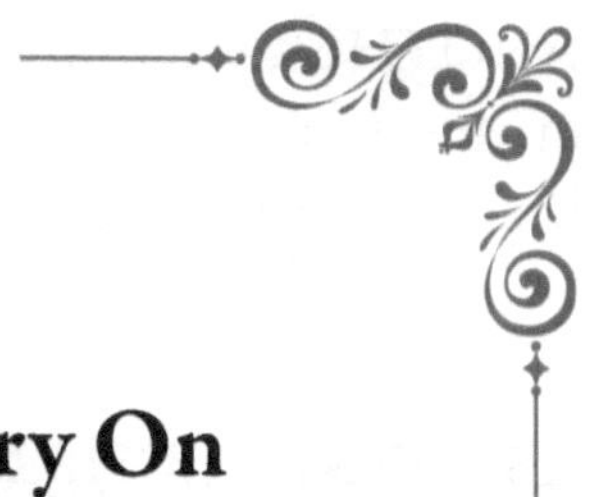

The Inside Story On Getting Pregnant

Opposed to conventional belief, pregnancy is not always an easy task to achieve. This is especially applicable to couples who tend to follow family planning and have set a target date on when they feel ready to have a child. It is rather important for everyone to understand that a number of factors can affect this goal.

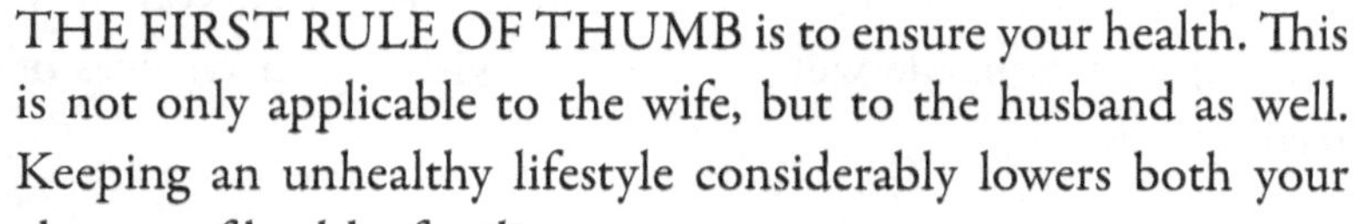

THE FIRST RULE OF THUMB is to ensure your health. This is not only applicable to the wife, but to the husband as well. Keeping an unhealthy lifestyle considerably lowers both your chances of healthy fertility.

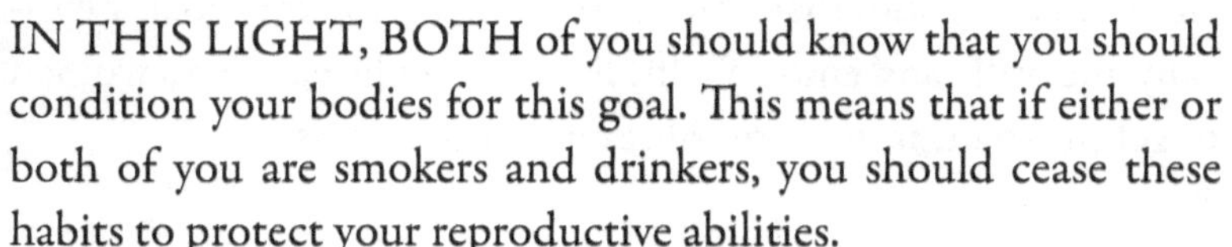

IN THIS LIGHT, BOTH of you should know that you should condition your bodies for this goal. This means that if either or both of you are smokers and drinkers, you should cease these habits to protect your reproductive abilities.

ANOTHER FACTOR TO CONSIDER is your weight. If you or your husband is on the heavier side, it is important that you begin to exercise and shed some of the extra pounds.

ABOVE ALL OTHER THINGS, having sex constantly is crucial. Think of it as a raffle entry. The more entries you have, the more chances you will gain to hit the jackpot.

MOST DOCTORS WILL LIKELY advise you to have sex at least once each day as you reach your day of ovulation. In technical terms, the sperm can survive for up to five days inside the fallopian tube before it dies.

CONSTANTLY HAVING SEX and ensuring that your husband ejaculates inside will provide you with higher chances of fertilization.

GETTING PREGNANT REQUIRES a lot of things. This includes making sure that you are both ready for this goal; physically, mentally and emotionally. It will never be easy for a woman to get pregnant if they are constantly under stress.

IF THEY EVER DO, THIS may also present a number of risks and complications to the entire term of the pregnancy. If both of you have a strong mindset, the more likely that your bodies will respond to reproduction and conception.

IN CASE THAT EITHER or both of begin to have qualms about the length of time that you have been trying to conceive, you should both see your family doctor.

IT IS NOT ALWAYS A necessity to consult a fertility clinic or professional. In often cases, simple vitamins, proper conditioning and minor lifestyle changes such as diet, habits and the like will serve as an essential tool in getting pregnant.

Essential Intercourse and Healthy Lifestyle Tips on How to Get Pregnant

Getting pregnant is most women's dream. They want to experience the joy of being a mother and so they will try their best to become one.

IT IS NORMALLY EASY to get pregnant if you are having a regular cycle and if luck hits you on your most recent intercourse. However, having an intercourse from time to time is not the answer for some women.

THIS IS BECAUSE THEIR sex life varies and their ovulation process is also different from each other. Learning how to get pregnant is more than just having intercourse.

THERE ARE SEVERAL THINGS to consider just before you start love-making. If your goal is to get pregnant that's why you are having sex, make sure that you are fertile.

YOUR EFFORT WILL GO to waste if you keep on having sex when you are not fertile. One way to determine if your body is ready for fertilization is by checking your cervical mucus. It has to be wet and slippery. It is your body's way to help sperms swim and fertilize an egg.

YOU WILL ALSO KNOW if you are possibly fertile if your basal body temperature (bbt) has just increased. A basal thermometer could help you with it. It is best to check for your bbt if you are relaxed.

THIS IS BECAUSE THE thermometer could accurately detect your body's temperature. When you keep on moving or have just finished cleaning your house, of course your body's temperature would be high, thus the thermometer's reading is going to be invalid. Your temperature is high not because you are fertile but because of your recent activity.

SINCE NOT ALL WOMEN have the same menstrual pattern, you have to be precise on the date of your ovulation period. One way on how to get pregnant is by keeping a chart or marking your calendar and see when do you usually have your first day.

IN THIS WAY, YOU CAN calculate your average ovulation period day which usually happens on the middle of the cycle. Normally, it is on the 14th day of a woman's 28-day cycle.

IF YOU ARE CERTAIN that you are fertile, have more intimate sex now. On the average, it could be thrice a week or everyday if you are sure that it's your ovulation week. Anyway, the sperm can stay longer for an average of three to five days.

AND WHILE YOU ARE BUSY with charting, body monitoring, and intercourse planning, don't forget that your lifestyle also plays an important role in helping your body to conceive.

CUT THE CAFFEINE INTAKE, get more folate, folic acid, and other vitamin supplements, don't get too exhausted and stressed, and quit (or stop for a while) smoking. Smoking can damage a part of your reproduction process.

YOUR PARTNER MUST ALSO be careful when doing his regular exercises. He must choose exercises that would not damage his groins. And finally, a doctor can always give you more advice on how to get pregnant that can suit you best.

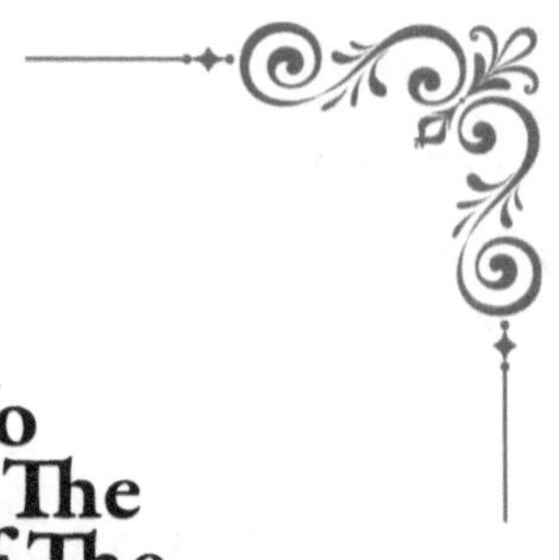

A Need To Understand The Functions Of The Reproductive System

When a couple begins their journey together, they dream of their future. They dream of moving in to a new home, in a new place where they will raise their children.

HOWEVER, WHEN EVERYTHING is being planned, some things just do not always come at the time that they were intended to. This is especially applicable when it comes to having children.

MOST COUPLES WHO HAVE been able to establish a 5-year or 10-year plan would often include family planning.

THIS MEANS THAT THEY will most likely be using birth control methods (natural or artificial) to ensure the timeline of being childfree. One factor to consider is that not everything that you have planned will go smoothly.

THIS IS WHY, IT IS important to know the facts on how to get pregnant. The first and most important thing to do is to understand how the human reproductive system really works.

IF YOU WOULD WANT TO ensure that your husband will be constantly fertile and can produce live and healthy sperm, there are a few things that you should need to know.

ONE OF THESE IS THE fact that their scrotum should ideally be at three to five degrees Fahrenheit below the normal body temperature.

THIS MEANS THAT THIS part of the body should constantly be cooler. When these are exposed to high temperatures, there are chances of temporary infertility. A urologist would be able to better explain these and more to you.

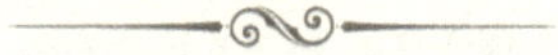

WHEN IT COMES TO WOMEN, knowing when you will ovulate will play a key role in successful egg fertilization. Most women (those with a precise 28-day monthly cycle) ovulate fourteen days after the onset of their monthly period.

HOWEVER, FOR OTHERS, determining this on their own can impose a challenge. The main reason for this to be essential is the fact that a fertilized egg only has a lifespan of 24 hours before it dies.

A GYNECOLOGIST WOULD be able to give you all the information that you will need for you to know when your ovulation will happen. They will also be able to tell you the steps that you can take to increase your chances of conception.

THE NEXT KEY TO GET you closer to pregnancy is to make love as often as you can. This should be especially applicable for the days before and during ovulation.

WHILE THE SPERM CAN survive for a number of days inside the fallopian tube, you should also remember that not all the sperm from the ejaculation comes out alive.

EACH TIME YOU MAKE love, you increase your chances of having a successful union between a healthy sperm and the egg. If you do this less frequently, you will decrease your chances adversely.

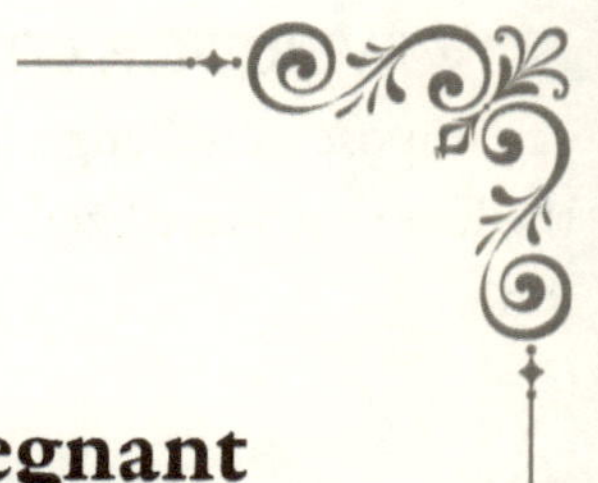

How to Get Pregnant by Learning About the Perfect Timing

Timing is very important when you want to get pregnant. You need to know when you are ovulating to ensure that there will be an egg ready for fertilization and take the form of another human being. If you have been searching for ways on how to get pregnant, understanding the perfect timing is a must.

THE BEST TIME TO TRY getting pregnant is when you are fertile. This is during your ovulation period when a mature ovum or egg is going to be available in the uterus for fertilization. Knowing when you are most fertile is very important because it's almost the same as knowing the best time to get pregnant.

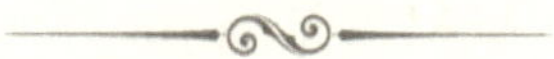

IF ALL THESE ARE QUITE new to you, here's a simple guide on how you can determine the perfect timing to conceive:

COUNTING THE DAYS – Counting the days in your menstrual cycle is one of the most effective ways in determining when it is best to make a baby.

TO DO THIS, YOU NEED to know when your next period is going to be. After computing it, count back from 12 to 16 days. The days in this period are when you are expected to ovulate. For women who have 28-day cycles, the best day to get pregnant is on the 14th day.

USING THIS METHOD IS easy especially for those who have regular menstrual cycles. There are ovulation calendars online which can help you plan out your fertile days even for months in advance.

Checking your cervical mucus – Your cervical mucus changes in texture and volume as your cycle progresses.

THIS MANIFESTS THAT your body's estrogen is rising. When the cervical mucus becomes clear, stretchy, and slippery in texture, this is the best time to have a baby.

NOW, YOU MAY BE WONDERING what the mucus has got to do with baby making. Well, a lot, actually. The mucus protects, nourishes, and speeds the sperm on the way up until it eventually meets the egg.

WHEN IT'S NOT AT ITS best, chances are it won't be as easy to have a baby.

MONITORING YOUR BASAL body temperature – Another indication of when it is best to get pregnant is the rise in your body temperature. After ovulating, your basal body temperature may increase by as much as 1. 6 degrees.

This shift is quite minimal so you won't really be aware of it, but you can measure it by using a basal thermometer. This increase in temperature is brought about by the increase of progesterone. Your progesterone level gets affected by ovulation.

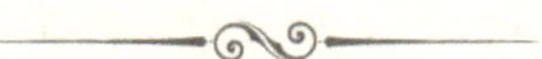

ANYWAY, THE BEST TIME to conceive is anytime between two and three days before your basal temperature reaches its peak. Of course, before being able to pinpoint when you are ovulating, you have to chart your basal temperature for several months.

THESE THREE ARE YOUR best tools in determining the perfect timing on when to have a baby. The circumstances on how to get pregnant may widely vary, but anyone who's trying to conceive should at least try these tools to make sure that their timing is right – before anything else.

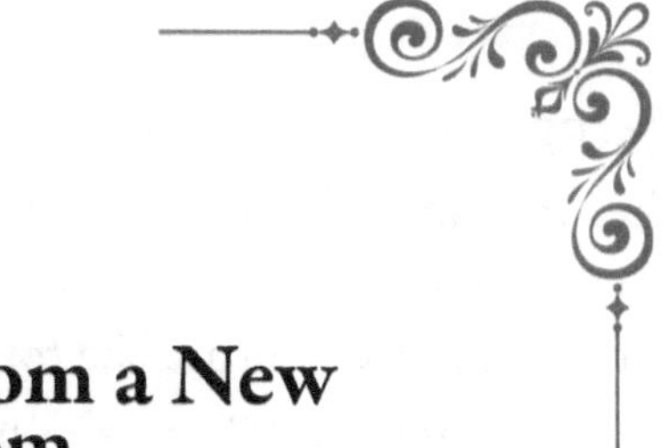

Advices from a New Mom

By the time you finish reading this, you will be all set to get pregnant. These how to get pregnant tips are well researched and tested. It is digested for you so you can easily follow the basics and will waste no time in trying to make a baby. So read on...

THROW AWAY YOUR BIRTH control pills – you should first and foremost discontinue taking these pills even months before getting pregnant as your body will still have to adjust to its ovulation cycles. This serves true with other birth control methods like using a patch or a ring.

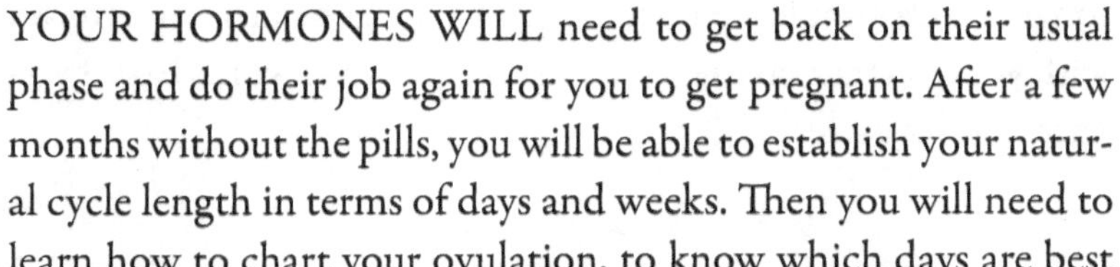

YOUR HORMONES WILL need to get back on their usual phase and do their job again for you to get pregnant. After a few months without the pills, you will be able to establish your natural cycle length in terms of days and weeks. Then you will need to learn how to chart your ovulation, to know which days are best to try to conceive a baby.

PREPARE YOUR BODY FOR your pregnancy – years of un-healthy eating habits and vices (if you have) will have to stop now. Ditch those junk foods and canned goods that have loads of preservatives and are bad for your health.

Kiss your cigarettes goodbye and give your drinking sessions a rest. It is important to get used to this kind of lifestyle because when you get pregnant, or even before you are, it is a must that your body is in tip top shape and will continue to be as you are getting ready for that baby you will carry for nine months.

KNOW WHEN YOU ARE FERTILE – this is the tricky part in the process of how to get pregnant because you will have to keep record of your monthly period. In the following months you will be able to see a pattern and this will help you determine your fertile days. Count 12 to 16 days backwards each month to know when you are likely to be ovulating based on your previous cycle.

IT SHOULD GIVE YOU an idea for the coming months as to when you should be ovulating, and by all means, do have sex with your partner on these days. This technique works best if you have regular cycles.

IF YOU HAVE AN IRREGULAR period, this may be a little tough to follow since you will not be able to determine the exact days or week you may be fertile. For women who have irregular menstrual cycles, you can use the BBT method (Basal Body Temperature).

YOU WILL HAVE TO GET your body temperature using a digital thermometer every morning before you get out of bed. Do this every day and after a few months you notice that when your body temperature shows a half-jump increase, this is the signal that you are ovulating. Take advantage of this phase and have great sex. It is more likely you will get pregnant if you know your fertile days.

SO THERE YOU HAVE IT. With these tips carefully observed and followed, it is very much possible that you will be blessed with your own bundle of joy. Soon enough, you will also be sharing different tips on how to get pregnant. Good luck!

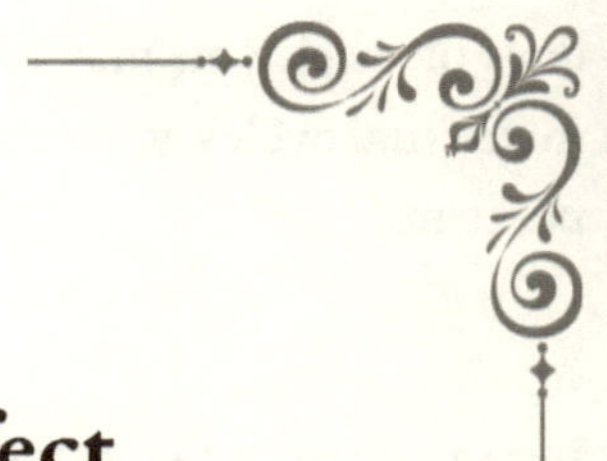

Have a Perfect Timing to Have an Intimate Intercourse

Getting pregnant may be easy for other women. Perhaps they are healthy enough to conceive or they are having a normal ovulation process. Maybe their partners could also produce healthy sperm cells.

HOWEVER, NOT ALL WOMEN have the same menstrual cycle, depending on their body's natural routine. If you've been waiting for months (or maybe a couple of years) to get pregnant and yet, there's no sign of life in your womb, it's better to consult some of the common advice on how to get pregnant.

SOMETIMES, THINKING that you are having enough sex is not enough to have a fertilized egg in your body.

INTERCOURSE IS THE main key to obtain sperm cells that will fertilize your egg. However, even if you have couple of sex in a month and there is no egg to be fertilized, it is useless. To increase your chances of getting pregnant, make sure you are having sex generously in a month.

THAT IS SEVERAL TIMES in a week. In this way, you could possibly be in your ovulation period when you have intercourse. A lucky sperm cell will be able to find an egg to fertilize. This will help you get the chance of being pregnant fast.

You may want to monitor your personal ovulation process. No one can help you detect your own fertility except for yourself. Try to get that basal thermometer and keep it beside your bed.

YOU MUST BE RELAXED when using that thermometer. You can get a more accurate reading if you will not be busy with other activities.

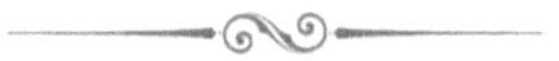

MOVING CAN INCREASE the temperature of your body. That will invalidate your thermometer's reading. Keeping an ovulation kit is also helpful in tracking your ovulation period.

IF YOU ARE AWARE THAT you must have intercourse before ovulation, then you know how to get pregnant fast. Check your calendar or your chart and see the time that your body will release an egg.

HAVE A GENEROUS SEX few days before that day to increase your chances of hitting the target. Since an egg can only survive for about one day, there must be sperm cells swarming around in the middle of your ovulation process. Besides, sperm cells can live up to around five days in search of an egg to fertilize.

YOU MAY HAVE READ FROM other sources that ovulation usually happens in the middle of your monthly cycle. But since there are some women who encounter it on an irregular basis (and you might be one of them), it is not highly advisable that you plan to have sex on the 14th day of the month. Know first when your ovulation will take place before start counting.

IT IS FINE TO FOLLOW the perfect timing to have intercourse based on some how to get pregnant tips but just don't end up having sex just to have a baby.

IT'S NOT ANYMORE RIGHT if sex turns out to be a couple's job or means on achieving something. Don't leave being intimate behind the picture. Enjoy lots of intercourse especially during the days that you think you are fertile.

Some Essential Tips To Consider When You Are Trying To Get Pregnant

Trends have shown that these days thanks to the kind of rushed up life that we lead, infertility has increased. This means that it is no longer as easy to get pregnant as it was in the good old days.

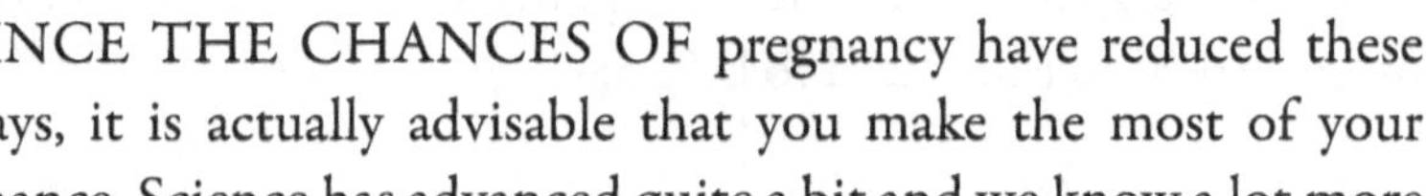

SINCE THE CHANCES OF pregnancy have reduced these days, it is actually advisable that you make the most of your chance. Science has advanced quite a bit and we know a lot more than our forefathers about the whole process of pregnancy.

THIS MEANS THAT WE can use this knowledge to increase our chances of getting pregnant. How to get pregnant in the quickest and most natural way?

THE FIRST IMPORTANT step for you is to consult a gynecologist. He or she would tell you all about your fertile periods and the steps that you might need to take to get pregnant.

YOU AND YOUR PARTNER might have to go through some tests to see if there might be any kind of inhibitor in your system. In case there is, then the doctor would suggest what to do to keep them from interfering. It is a smart move to calculate your exact ovulation timing. The physician would guide you on how to go about it. You can also work out the calculation yourself with an ovulation calculator. In case you do not trust this calculator you could double check with the help of a basal body thermometer.

ENSURE THAT YOU ARE having regular unprotected intercourse during this time. The average life span of a sperm in the uterus has been calculated to be 2 days.

THIS MEANS THAT YOU can increase your chances of pregnancy by having regular unprotected sex around 2 or more days before actual ovulation. It is even advisable that you lie down a few minuets after intercourse.

THIS KEEPS THE SEMEN in the body for some time, allowing it to reach the uterus. In case you take birth control pills on a regular basis, your body would need some time to get adjusted to the absence of birth control. This means that it would take your body around 3 months to be ready to conceive after you are off birth control.

YOU WOULD EVEN NEED to modify your diet. Try eating as healthy as possible. Give up on any unhealthy habit that you might have. In case you are into a habit of smoking and drinking, you would need to give it up soon. These interfere with the fertility of the body. Some studies have even shown that caffeine is not good for the reproductive health of the body. It would be no harm indeed to give up on the caffeine for the next few days.

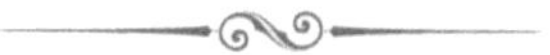

KEEP THE STRESS LEVEL as low as possible. In fact it has been seen that stress releases certain hormones in the body which interfere with the productivity of the body.

GIVE YOURSELF SOME time. You will not get pregnant immediately. Do not get impatient in case you are not pregnant within the next 6 months. It will happen slowly and steadily.

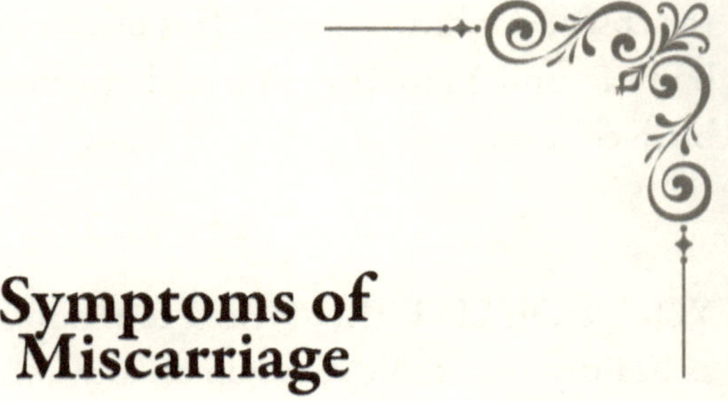

Symptoms of Miscarriage

Learn the signs and symptoms that may indicate miscarriage. No matter when it happens, the miscarriage is never an easy experience.

YOU SHOULD ALSO REMEMBER that in most cases, a miscarriage will have no influence on the future design of another child, and most women will have the opportunity to give birth later.

HOW TO DETECT A MISCARRIAGE?

IF YOU ARE STILL IN the stage called early pregnancy (less than 2 ½ months), the most common sign is a loss of blood and broken. Note that small losses of blood are quite normal and can happen at a slight detachment of the placenta.

THIS IS WHY IT IS ALWAYS necessary that you go see your doctor after the bleeding. Another sign of miscarriage can be deflating the breasts or the sudden stop vomiting morning.

IF YOU ARE IN THE ADVANCED stage of pregnancy (fourth or fifth month), the cervix is usually open and violent contractions are felt. You will also have significant blood loss and an amniotic fluid flow.

The main causes of miscarriage

During the early miscarriage, miscarriage is usually caused by the non-viability of the embryo. Indeed, at this stage, you are not wearing an egg and if a malfunction is detected by the chromosome body, it will naturally stop the process of pregnancy, the embryo not being able to develop properly.

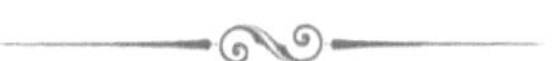

IT CAN ALSO BE AN EMPTY egg, which the embryo will not develop only after fertilization, for various reasons.

WHEN MISCARRIAGE LATER (after 2 ½ months), the problem is usually mechanical in nature. It may be a problem with the cervix, which opens with each contraction for do not close when he must remain flexible and strong.

THIS KIND OF PROBLEM is usually solved before the next pregnancy what is called a cerclage cervical. Perhaps you have a viral infection, mainly vaginosis or listeriosis, caused by ingestion of contaminated dairy products.

IT MAY BE THAT YOUR uterus is obviously too narrow for the developing embryo. To remedy this problem, surgery is sometimes necessary to pregnancies and type are generally well monitored.

MAKE SEVERAL CONSECUTIVE miscarriages

AFTER THREE CONSECUTIVE miscarriages, it is called recurrent miscarriage. From this point on, the doctor will do a complete examination of the female body and the human gene to detect the cause of these miscarriages.

YOU SHOULD KNOW THIS because once discovered, most problems can be fixed either by surgery or by taking specific drugs. Remember also that the miscarriage is never the fault of the surrogate mother but is usually associated with accident of nature.

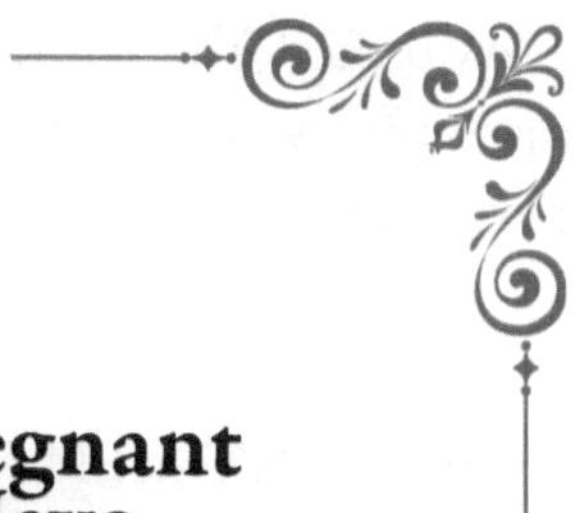

How to Get Pregnant When You Have Polycystic Ovarian Disease

Women who are suffering from polycystic ovarian syndrome otherwise known as PCOS may have a harder time getting pregnant. The disease is one of the main causes of infertility among women, thus, having it could be detrimental to the plans of conception.

THE ABSOLUTE CURE FOR PCOS is still unknown. However, the good thing is that there's really no need to give up the quest on how to get pregnant. Women with PCOS can conceive provided that they get the right treatment.

ALTHOUGH THE NUMBER of women who are having a hard time conceiving due to PCOS is not alarming yet, it is undeniable that the situation can be very frustrating to those who are in it.

HAVING THE DISEASE can cause numerous problems and discomforts. They may range from delayed conception to complications with pregnancy to increased risk of miscarriages.

IN SOME WOMEN, THE early symptoms of PCOS are their erratic and irregular periods. They will have it this month and not have it for three months. Sometimes, they don't have periods at all. Although this may primarily sound convenient, it spells big trouble among couples who can't wait to start a family and welcome a new addition in their home.

COMMONLY, WOMEN WHO have PCOS have less than 9 periods in a frame of one year. However, there are also cases when PCOS sufferers have regular periods but they do not ovulate every time, or in some cases, they do not ovulate at all.

IF YOU HAVE PCOS AND you wish to get pregnant, the way to deal with your problem is to go through infertility treatments. The most popular way that doctors suggest is by taking medications.

THE MEDICATIONS ARE expected to work by encouraging ovulation. This method generally works and can significantly increase your chances of being fertile and eventually getting pregnant.

IF MEDICATIONS DON'T seem to work, the next common step is the use of hormones. Just like the medications, hormones are expected to stimulate ovulation. There is also this surgical procedure called "ovarian drilling" which involves drilling small holes in the ovaries using a laser.

THE PROCEDURE MAY HELP in restoring ovulation, or at least promote the efficacy of the medications by stimulating the ovaries to respond to them.

When both treatments fail, there is a more radical option for a more-than-willing couple. The procedure is called In Vitro Fertilization or IVF.

THIS IS WHEN THE EMBRYO is injected into the woman's uterus where it is expected to grow in stages just as it would if it were successfully formed in the conventional way. IVF can be very costly and not many people can afford them. However, when all else failed, this may be the best option.

DEALING WITH THE ISSUE of how to get pregnant may be a bit more challenging to women with PCOS, however, it is no reason to lose hope or give up. It's not the end of the world. Many PCOS sufferers eventually had babies. If they did, so can you.

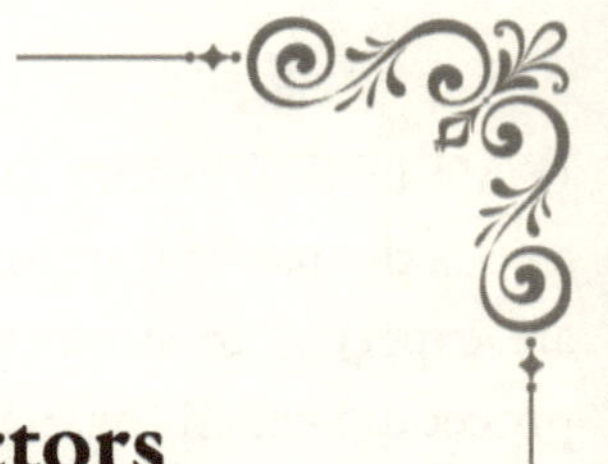

Common Factors Which Affect Female Fertility

I nfertility is when a person is unable to conceive a baby after a year or more of trying. If you are infertile, it is best to consult a fertility doctor to know of your best options in dealing with the condition.

THERE ARE MANY FACTORS which affect fertility. As fertility problems are a little more often on the woman's side, let us discuss here what affects the female fertility.

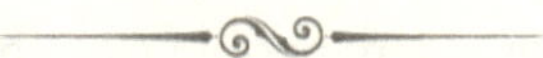

THE PRIMARY FACTOR that influences a woman's fertility is her age. As ovaries deteriorate as a woman grows old, there is really a certain period when it is best to get pregnant. This period is between 23 and 31 years old.

SOME CAN STILL MANAGE well till 35. However, anywhere beyond this age may be difficult because a significant decrease in fertility happens during this time onwards.

ANOTHER REASON FOR infertility is ovulation problems due to hormonal imbalances. When there is a hormonal disorder in a woman's system, she could experience different abnormalities such as having empty follicles, their failure, or their being ruptured. The rhythm of the hormones is very crucial. Even just a slight imbalance in it may trigger an ovulation problem.

IN THE US, THERE'S a condition that is prevalent among women who are having troubles getting pregnant. It is called Polycystic Ovarian Syndrome or PCOS.

THIS CONDITION IS TYPIFIED by having high levels of androgen and testosterone (male hormones) that result in the ability of the reproductive system of a woman to produce mature eggs. Women who have PCOS often experience acne breakout and increase in facial hairs.

There is also a disease called Pelvic Inflammatory Disease or PID. This is another factor why a woman fails to conceive. This disease involves a range of infections which affect the reproductive organs.

FOR INSTANCE, THERE'S salpingitis or the infection in the fallopian tubes. This infection is quite a frequent cause of infertility in females. When there's recurrent infection, it can lead to tubal damages.

ANOTHER CONDITION WHICH is a common cause of infertility in women is endometriosis. This is when some fragments of the endometrial lining are lodged in other pelvic areas. This may lead to development of cysts that can hinder pregnancy.

THERE ARE INDEED QUITE a number of conditions that may affect the ability of a woman to get pregnant. More often, the doctor can prescribe some medications that can help correct the imbalances and malfunctions; although there isn't really any guarantee as to when the woman being treated could eventually conceive.

IF YOU HAVE BEEN TRYING to have a baby for sometime but luck hasn't come yet, the best thing to do is consult a doctor as soon as possible. He or she can help pinpoint the problem and guide you towards the best solution in dealing with it.

HAVING A BABY IS A big thing. When the going gets tough, tell yourself that perhaps the reason why you don't have a baby yet is because there are bigger things you need to cover aside from just knowing how to get pregnant. Practice more patience. The baby will eventually come.

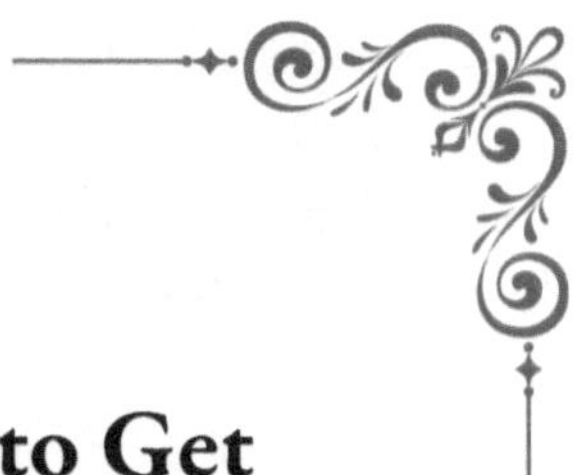

The Safest Way to Get Pregnant

There are two types of women – one who can get pregnant without a sweat and one who is experiencing difficulties in conceiving. Some women are lucky to get pregnant without even trying. On the other hand, there are some women who cannot conceive despite the fact that they have been trying to get pregnant.

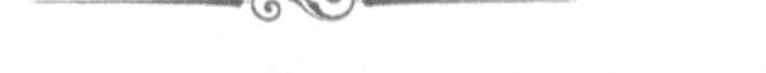

BELOW ARE TIPS ON HOW to get pregnant the safest way that will surely help you solve your dilemma.

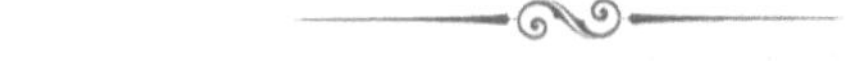

REMOVE THE IDEA THAT you will be able to get pregnant once you take a lot of sex. It is not that way. There are only limited days that you can get pregnant.

Why? Because there are only a few days that a woman is fertile or it is at its peak. It means that roughly 25 percent is your only chance of getting pregnant each month.

YOU HAVE TO KNOW PROPER timing when conceiving. An ideal 28 day cycle's ovulation is on the 14th day. But not all women have the perfect cycle. Some has longer and some has shorter cycles. Some do not ovulate on the halfway point.

IT'S COMMON THAT A woman may ovulate on the 13h, 14th, 15th or 16th. Ovulation changes every month. If you will use this as your means of identifying your ovulation period, you better make a chart of your menstruation cycle first for a couple of months. Jut down the dates for you to know the trend of your cycle.

GET YOUR BASAL TEMPERATURE and chart the results. Do this for a couple of months in order for you to know how to predict when are you ovulating. Take your temperature every morning before doing anything.

REMEMBER THAT YOU HAVE to let the sperm "waiting" for the egg cell to be released. So the best time to have contact is before ovulation period. Egg cell last only for abut 12 to 24 hours while sperm cell can last up to three to five days.

DO NOT USE STANDING and sitting sexual positions when making love because it has shallow penetration. Instead, use rear-entry, side by side and missionary sexual positions to have dipper penetration. The goal is to have the sperm cell swim near the cervix which can be done by having the right sexual positions.

ON THE DAY YOU DECIDED to get pregnant, stop taking any pills. It takes time to go back to your regular menstrual cycle.

EAT FOODS THAT ARE rich in folic acid and vitamins C. Avoid foods that are rich in carbohydrates and trans fat.

The tips listed above on how to get pregnant the safest way have been tested by many couples who were having a hard time in getting pregnant.

THE COUPLES WHO HAVE done the tips are now enjoying their much desired blessing – having a baby. So what are you waiting for? Try now the tips and be one of the couples who became successful in getting pregnant.

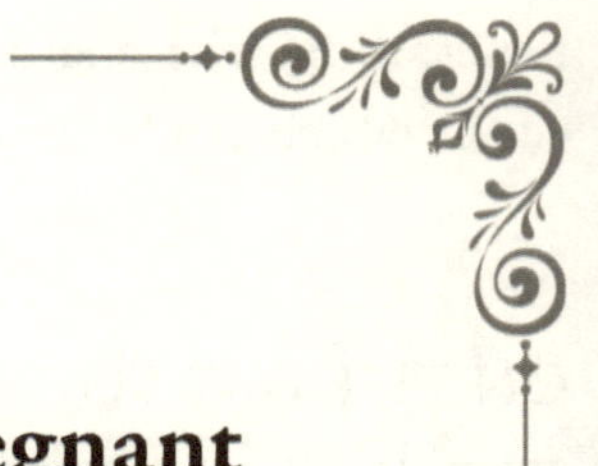

How to Get Pregnant with Assisted Reproductive Techniques

Have you been trying too long to get pregnant? Are you over 35 and are worrying that you might be running out of time? Are you tired of listening to people's advice on how to get pregnant while none of these advices seem to work for you?

IF YOU HAVE BEEN TRYING unprotected sexual intercourse for more than 2 years at a stretch then you actually might be having fertility problems.

OF COURSE THAT DOES not mean that all is lost. These days there are a lot of couples who actually face the problems of infertility because of the stress and strain that is so closely associated with today's lifestyle.

THAT IS WHY THERE ARE a number of new techniques developed by the medical community to help you get pregnant. It

50

must be understood, that when a couple fails to have a child, it is because either one of the partners of both of the might be facing problems of impotency.

MEDICAL COMMUNITY HAS new methods called the assisted reproductive treatments where this can be sought to be corrected. So if you are wondering on how to get pregnant with the help of the medical community, there are loads of methods that could be used by you.

FIRST OF ALL GET YOURSELF diagnosed. There are different approaches of dealing with infertility depending on whom the problem lies with. The male partner often shows low sperm count. Because of the low sperm count there are not enough sperms which enter the female's body for fertilisation. So how to get pregnant if that is where the problem lies?

THE ANSWER LIES IN artificial insemination. What the clinics do is pick up the male partner's sperm and place it in the womb of the female artificially. This leads to conception and thus pregnancy.

OFTEN IT HAS BEEN SEEN that the male sperm count is just as it should be and the health of the sperms are fine as well. Yet the fertilisation does not happen. This is because the uterus of the woman is too weak for fertilisation.

HOW TO GET PREGNANT in such a situation? The answer lies in surrogacy. Here there is a third woman who permits to let her womb out. The male's sperm and female's egg is extracted out of the body and is artificially placed into this womb. However, this is a hell of an expensive procedure and therefore not a much desired one as well.

There are often certain situations when both the male and the female partner might be suffering from the qualms of impotency. How to get pregnant in such a situation?

IN VITRO FERTILIZATION is one of the most desired methods that are adopted in such a scenario. Here the egg and the sperm are extracted from the bodies and fertilised in a test tube.

ONCE FERTILISATION is complete, the fertilized egg is put back into the womb of the woman ready for growth and nourishment. In case you are facing problems in conceiving, you can actually take the assistance of the medical community and get pregnant.

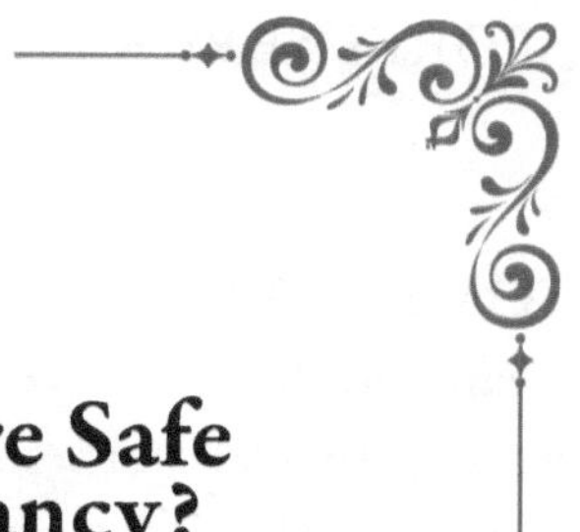

What Sports are Safe During Pregnancy?

Choose your sports carefully during pregnancy. You are pregnant and you are rather sporty nature. You're probably wondering if you can still perform an activity.

SOME ACTIVITIES PUT you at greater risk for injury than others. Everything depends on the sports considered, your training and your health. This brings benefits and relaxes you, if you do not force it and it is a gentle practice.

WHY GO TO THE GYM?

A PRIORI, YOU HAVE no reason to quit a sport daily if it is not aggressive and you are in good health . Instead it can be a lovely time for you and your baby . You will be more relaxed and you will accompany your body changing. Choose a sport for that smooth.

SPORTS AT RISK FOR pregnant women

SOME SPORTS ARE TO be avoided, especially if they are violent and they will face a fall or trauma of any kind. Even if you are experienced in these disciplines, it is strongly recommended to the ski , the riding or climbing because the risk of falling is too great.

ATHLETICS SHOULD BE discontinued at the end of the second month of pregnancy . In general, sports team or battle where shocks are frequent, should not be practiced.

Sports recommended during pregnancy

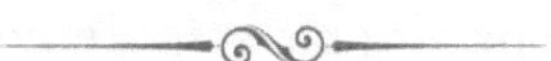

WALKING: FOR ALL MOMS , walking is a great way to move. It is a good option if you stop an activity incompatible with your pregnancy or you're not athletic.

SWIMMING: WHETHER YOU are a good or a bad swimmer, the swimming or water aerobics is the best sport during pregnancy with walking. In addition to its calming, improve your breathing which helps you during childbirth .

YOU ALSO WORK YOUR perineum , and you strengthen your muscles. However, avoid diving into water that is too cold.

Yoga: This is both a sports and a good preparation for the birth .

The benefits are almost identical to those of swimming .

Pilates: what sports can relieve some pain associated with pregnancy and better control his breathing.

REMEMBER YOU CONTROL

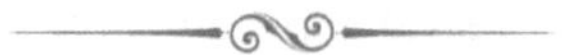

PRACTICE A SPORTS YES but you leaving. It does not make you more tired. You must know your limits. Any excess can be dangerous because it can result in a risk of hypoxia (lack of oxygen).

YOU SHOULD ALSO CHECK your heart rate, take your pulse for 15 minutes and multiply by four to get the score on a minute. Note that in early pregnancy , you get winded faster and your pulse is faster.

Weight Gain During Pregnancy

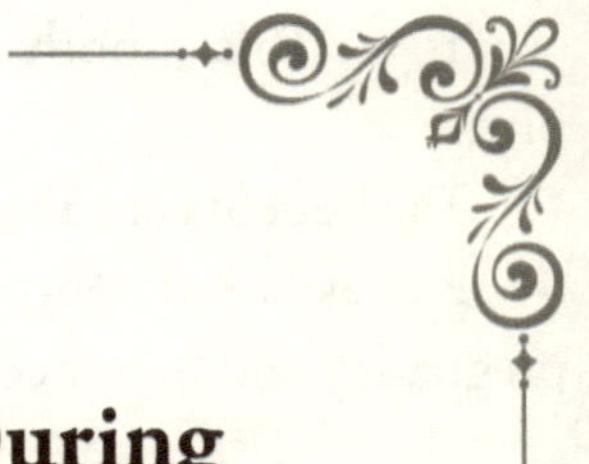

There are numerous false truths circulating on weight gain through pregnancy. Difficult to differentiate amid true and false. Once past the first few months the weight gain is usually well controlled.

COMES TO THE FULLNESS that sometimes goes to some carelessness food. So where should he remain vigilant and where can we make concessions of a nutritional point of view?

TO CLARIFY THE IDEAS are reported on 10 myths about weight, the pounds and pregnancy.

1. Since I'm pregnant, I feel I have more hunger than before.

THAT IS CORRECT. DURING pregnancy, hormones cause a significant increase in appetite grow. You will certainly tend to increase more or less the size of your food intake, even without you noticing.

2. DURING PREGNANCY, you must eat for two.

NO, WE DO NOT EAT FOR two during pregnancy. However, we eat better, we have paid more attention to the contributions necessary for the mom and baby ! Your appetite should gradually regulate energy intake as you need.

3. SPEAKER, WE TAKE 1 kg per month.

This is incorrect. If weight gain actually follows a curve mechanically lift the weight gained is not even following the term of pregnancy.

IN THE FIRST QUARTER

Weight gain is low. Some women may even lose weight at the beginning when they have nausea or vomiting.

IN THE SECOND QUARTER

It accelerates! It was during the second quarter than mothers feel shots craving or the famous "wants" (sometimes disgust). Do not deprive yourself, but beware of snacks: better split meals (four or five small meals) and not throw it on the sweet. In the sixth month, it is taking 6 kilos, not less.

If you have one or two extra pounds, it is not very serious. If you see your weight curve to fly, talk to your doctor.

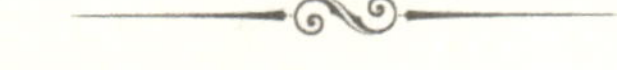

IN THE THIRD QUARTER

IT IS RECOGNIZED THAT weight gain is now 1 kilo to 1.5 kilo per month, a total weight gain in late pregnancy 9 kg to 12 kg. This weight gain is perfect for mom and baby.

CAREFUL THE LAST FEW weeks are the most treacherous: You are stopped, quite inactive and food drives are sometimes difficult or impossible to curb. Weight gain in recent weeks may be spectacular, but without starving yourself, stay vigilant!

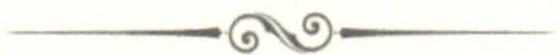

4. THE DISTRIBUTION of weight is half to the mother, the other half to the baby.

This is false. Took the pounds will benefit differently to mother and baby.

For baby

3 to 4 kg.

For the mother:

Uterus: 900 g

Placenta : 500g

Breast : 400g

Blood volume: 1.5 kg

Lipid reserves: 2 to 3 kg

Water Retention: 2 kg

Please note: Some of pounds used to establish a reserve of fat that will be used when breastfeeding .

5 – Weight gain can be very different from one woman to another.

Indeed, all women are different. And each live weight gain during pregnancy differently. However, there are variables for estimating the weight gain as desirable women.

TO ESTIMATE THIS WEIGHT gain, it is necessary to refer to the body mass index (BMI) before pregnancy calculated according to the formula of Lorenz. This is the ratio between weight and height in meters squared.

To calculate: (size -100) – (-150 size) / 2.5.

6. I see that I took too much weight, I can make up my birth plan.

FALSE. AVOID DIETS during pregnancy, they are a source of failures and frustrations. If you see that you have taken too much weight, talk to your doctor who will be better able to give you good advice and you specify foods that should not be removed from your diet.

Remember that you eat for you but also for your little baby changing.

7. I HAVE TO FIGHT against my desires.

Absolutely not! Do you dream of chocolate or candies, caramels or friezes sugar? Allow yourself the simple pleasures sometimes ... Know grant you good times while remaining reasonable. These desires are not too whims and try to resist, you could be back on something else sometimes worse.

8. Even if I do not carry much weight, you should be wary of stretch marks.

IN FACT, IF YOU MAGNIFY less risk of stretch marks are reduced. However, other factors are involved in the formation of these unsightly marks. Cortisol (pregnancy hormone) can for example result from the start of pregnancy. The youthful skin and firmness are also factors that increase the risk of developing stretch marks: take care of your skin.

9. MEDICALLY, THERE is no risk to gain weight during pregnancy.

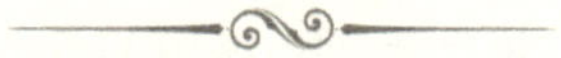

THIS IS FALSE. IT IS quite normal to gain weight during pregnancy but avoid excess. Not only because the extra pounds will be difficult to lose after the birth and can affect your mood, morale and encourage the baby blues .

IN ADDITION, WEIGHT gain is too important a factor in the genesis of gestational diabetes . Do not forget that a few extra pounds during your pregnancy, you may tire more quickly and suffer from back pain.

10. IF I WERE OVERWEIGHT before my pregnancy, it makes it a little more complicated.

INDEED, OVERWEIGHT complicates the advent of pregnancy has an effect on the hormonal balance and cycles; being frequently synonymous with problems of ovulation and reducing the effectiveness of the LDCs . In addition, overweight before pregnancy predisposes the mother- in:

Risk of false-layer higher in the first quarter.

More problems of high blood pressure.

A high risk of gestational diabetes .

A cesarean section rate more frequently.

Good news is that, despite a last belief, overweight before pregnancy has no influence on the risk of preterm baby.

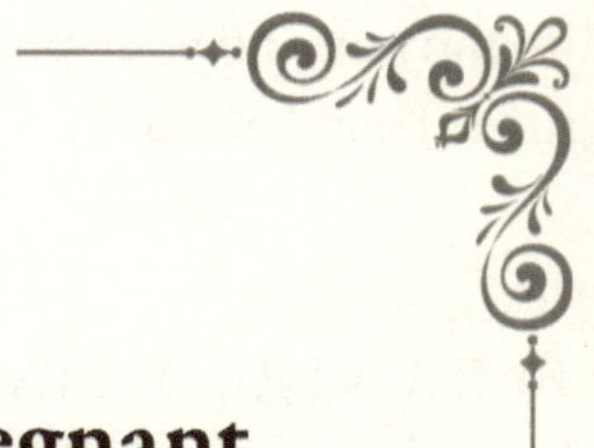

How to Get Pregnant With Twin

For a family, a very special present is to get pregnant with twins. Visualize that you need to have a dual preparation to receive or welcome your two little infants simultaneously.

AND ALSO, MORE CARE and attention must be given to the pregnant mommy. Getting twins must be a sort of surprise that can be admitted by a partner in different manners.

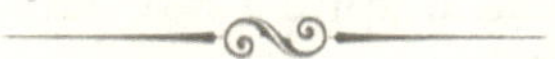

IF THE GREATER PART of couples admits this expensive gift with cheerfulness and happiness, there are some other partners who admit this with apprehension and hesitation.

WITHOUT DOUBT, THERE are lots of aspects to be measured in terms of getting pregnant with twins as well as raising two kids all at once.

PHYSICAL HEALTH AND financial capability are the most significant factors to be considered. You could experience a higher danger and possibility of complications like preeclampsia and premature birth.

ALSO, YOU MIGHT THINK that your expenses will almost two times if raising two kids which is the main issue of almost every couple. But, you might be among those partners who desire to have twins and are attempting hard to get it.

IT IS POSSIBLE BUT it is not very easy. Try to understand that there are several hereditary aspects that might affect your attempt getting twins.

A LOT OF STUDIES HAVE shown that pregnancy for twins has a hereditary basis. Especially, fraternal twinning happens if 2 diverse eggs are fertilized by 2 diverse sperm cells all at once to form 2 zygotes thus fraternal twins are also known as non-identical twins or dizygotic twins.

HOWEVER, THE KEY ASPECT for this fraternal twin to occur which is the capability to discharge more than a single egg, lies just in the mother. There's no proof that the factor of the father comes into responsibility in this system.

ALTERNATIVELY, IT LOOKS that identical twinning or monozygotic is not controlled by a hereditary aspect. Some folks will possibly inform you that breastfeeding while you are pregnant can gain the possibilities having twins.

MOREOVER, IT'S BELIEVED and might be backed up by several researches that to get pregnant in mature age is already dangerous, the more when you have to consider twins.

It's stated that ovulation turns into quicker at that age. In addition to this, there is a suggestion according to a study by a dependable organization to gain your BMI or known as Body Mass Index to thirty or higher is superior which signifies that you must be considered as overweight. If your Body Mass Index is 25, you are considered as obese already.

AS YOU MIGHT HAVE THE perceptive that obese or overweight are most possible to experience from infertility, in that way this issue must be a simplified.

AS A RESULT, THE GREAT technique if you really want twins or desire to best way to get pregnant with twins is to visit your obstetrician or physician.

WITHOUT DOUBT, SHE or he will give you the best or consistent information on this matter. And also, you can simplify the above mentioned issues.

The Causes of Female Infertility

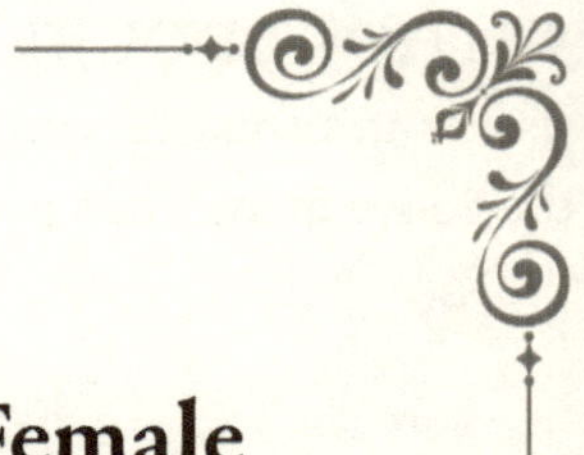

What Causes Female Infertility? Infertility is the inability of a couple to become pregnant after 12 months of unprotected intercourse. There are many factors to female infertility.

WITH SO MANY POTENTIAL causes, facing female infertility can be both stressful and confusing. Learn about the causes of female infertility and investigate the various causes in infertility in women.

OVARIAN CAPRICIOUS disrupt ovulation

IN SOME WOMEN, THE presence of ovarian microcysts or malfunction of the pituitary and hypothalamus glands (glands in the brain that release the female hormones) inhibit the release of an egg from the ovaries.

IT IS IMPOSSIBLE TO cross the road to the sperm. To treat these disorders of ovulation , drug treatment (ovarian stimulation) can be effective, provided it is moderate (risk of hyperstimulation) and monitored by a physician. Radiotherapy or chemotherapy treatments indicated for cancer, can also damage the ovaries.

TUBAL OBSTRUCTIONS

The fallopian tubes of – which passes through the egg to reach the uterus – can become clogged. This closure of the fallopian tubes is the result of salpingitis (200 000 new cases each year in France). This infection of the fallopian tubes is caused by sexually transmitted bacteria.

AN ABNORMAL ENDOMETRIUM: endometriosis

THE ENDOMETRIUM – OR endometrium – may pose some problems in the design if it is not right consistency. The uterine lining may be too thin and thus prevents the embryo clinging, or, conversely, too exuberant.

IN THIS CASE, DOCTORS speak of endometriosis . This disorder of the uterine lining is manifested by the presence of endometrium on the ovaries, fallopian tubes, bladder and even the intestines!

Women who are infected have rules generally very painful and 30-40% of them difficult to become pregnant. To treat endometriosis, two methods: hormone therapy or surgery.

UTERUS INHOSPITABLE

WHEN THE SPERM MET the egg in the uterus , the party is not over yet! Sometimes the egg fails to implant in the uterus due to a defect or the presence of fibroids or polyps in the uterus. Sometimes it's the mucus secreted by the cervix, which is necessary to allow the passage of sperm, which is inadequate or nonexistent. A simple hormone therapy may be offered to increase the secretion of these glands.

LIFESTYLE PLAYS ON fertility

THERE IS NO SECRET, "wanting a baby" rhymes with "healthy" ...! The tobacco , alcohol, stress, obesity or, conversely, a diet too restrictive, are all harmful to the fertility of men and women. It is striking and rather frightening to see that the sperm were much richer and mobile in the years 70-80 today! It is therefore important to have a healthy lifestyle to boost fertility

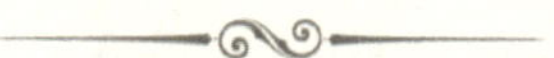

OTHER THAN THE COMMON causes mentioned above, infertility can occur due to vast number of medical and surgical abnormalities. In many cases, it may be due to abnormalities in both the partners to some extent. Some of the causes include:

CONGENITAL ABNORMALITIES, such as septate uterus, unicornuate uterus

Abnormalities of Cervical mucus

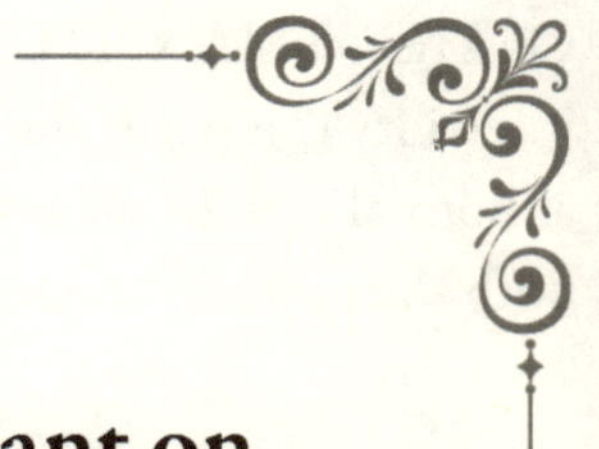

Can I get pregnant on my period

Asking the question "can I get pregnant on my period" is something that many people have done for a really long time.

THIS IS OFTEN A QUESTION that many people will answer with a very firm "no" because they have a few beliefs that might actually be incorrect.

THIS ARTICLE WILL HIGHLIGHT the main belief that most individuals have and it will also discuss the truth related to the age old question of "can I get pregnant on my period"?

ONE OF THE MAIN REASONS why people will say no when others ask "can I get pregnant on my period" is because they fully understand that when a woman has her period she is ridding her body of the egg that needs to be fertilized by the sperm in order for pregnancy to occur in the first place.

THEREFORE, IF THERE is no egg, then there is no pregnancy. This does sound legitimate and it does make sense to an extent.

What these people do not think about is the fact that sperm do not die within hours of sexual intercourse. So, let us take some time to look at that fact now.

When you are asked "can I get pregnant on my period" there are many factors that need to be taken into consideration. First of all, it is always great idea to realize that sperm can live within the body for several days. That means that if you were not ovulating on the day that you had sexual intercourse you can still become pregnant.

You really need to spend some time thinking about your body. You will need to learn when you ovulate. This will help you determine if having sex on your period is really safe.

It is often believed that most women will ovulate around day 14 of their cycle. This is true if the female is on a 28 day cycle but not all women are.

WITH THAT BEING SAID, it will be very important to take the time to study your body and the signs of ovulation in order to identify when you are ovulating.

THIS CAN ALSO BE DONE by learning how long your cycle is. It may be a 32 day cycle. That does not mean that there is anything wrong with you, or that you are not ovulating at all, but it can help you identify when conception is more likely to happen for you and your partner.

THERE ARE SOME INDIVIDUALS that will find out that they are ovulating a few short days after they have had their period.

THAT MEANS THAT IF couple had sex while the female was on her period the sperm could survive until the egg is released into the fallopian tube. At this time pregnancy could be very possible. Women and men alike need to understand this in order to realize that they can become pregnant if they make the decision to have sex while the woman is on her period.

EVERYONE KNOWS THAT teens are becoming more and more sexually active and they are also becoming sexually active at a much younger age now than they were before.

MANY OF THESE TEENS often think that they are not able to become pregnant when they have sex on their period. It is easy to see from this brief article that the truth of the matter is that they can get pregnant if they engage in sexual intercourse when they are on their period.

BECAUSE OF THIS, TEENS need to be educated fully on this topic. It is much better for them to have all of the facts rather than entering into this act blindly and ending up pregnant.

IT CAN BE VERY DIFFICULT for adolescents to understand their bodies and how pregnancy works. After all, just think about how difficult it can be for adults to understand this process and how it works.

"CAN I GET PREGNANT on my period" is a good question to ask but it also has a number of different answers when you think about it. There are so many different factors to consider and leaving out just one of those factors could result in an unwanted pregnancy. It is always best to use protection or to avoid sex until marriage is a pregnancy is not planned.

www.ingramcontent.com/pod-product-compliance
Lightning Source LLC
Chambersburg PA
CBHW031325250726
48656CB00005B/1973